An Editor's Corner

Reflections On
How Dentistry is Changing

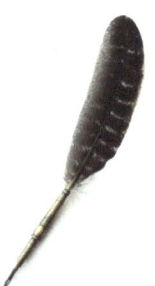

by
Neil Stewart McLeod

An Editor's Corner

Reflections On How Dentistry is Changing

by
Neil Stewart McLeod

An Editor's Corner
Reproduction and copying of this book by any means is encouraged. The primary material was all originally published in the "the Explorer" the newsletter for the Los Angeles Dental Society.
Neil Stewart McLeod, Los Angeles, California.

By the same author

A Ship In A Bottle
One for the Pot
The Clan Remembers
Pure Whimsy
The Aching Heart
The Thorn With Me
My Silver Box
When the Spirit Moves
A Cartload of Stories
The Persimmon Tree
Songs and Poems of Frances McLeod
The Illustrated Address to A Haggis
Letters From A Scottish Chief
Dental Ditties
Another Cuppa
Nearly Jewish

ISBN-13: 978-1720369295

Contents

An Introduction 3

What's In A Word 4

The Oldest Profession... 6

Not The First ... Nor Yet The Last 8

Capitalizing on Current News 10

Final Impressions - The End Of An Era? 14

Is Digital Better 16

Don't Rush To Brush 18

Giving In To Market Pressure 22

Are You Making The Up-Grade 24

Brain Wave 27

Sad or Sorry - Dental Service Organizations - a euphemism 29

Dedication
for my daughter in law
Bilyana
entering the profession

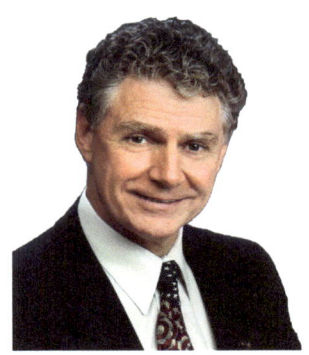

An Introduction

For two years, from 2015 - 2017, I have had the privilege of serving as "editor" of *Explorer*, the newsletter for the Los Angeles Dental Society. I put the word editor in quotation marks because the real work of overseeing the production and conning through the content fell on the shoulders of Teresa Chien, the Executive Director, and her staff. My task was to come up with something interesting and pithy that was topical that might catch the reader's attention, and try to do as good a job as my predecessors like Dr. Kenneth Jacobs. Running through these short articles is an appeal to our profession to keep up to date and yet exercise caution as we do so. We have an amazing history being responsible for the introduction of fine miniaturized drills, anesthesia implantology and exquisite ceramic prosthetic replacements. Here then are the eleven articles that were published as the Editor's Corner. The opportunity to expand content and add a poem was irresistible.

Neil Stewart McLeod, BDS, LDS RCS, DDS

Los Angeles, California, 2017

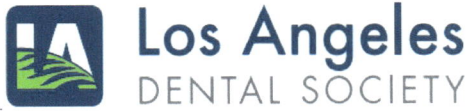

WHAT'S IN A WORD

The word "doctor" means teacher, it is derived from the Latin root "dictus" to proclaim or speak and "docere" to teach. Implicit in the title is the trusted responsibility to teach our patients what their treatment options are so that they can make an informed decision on what care they will acquiesce to receive from our hands. It is incidental that we also provide the care we have recommended, but first and foremost our patients trust us to give them sound advice that is honest.

As dentists we have come a long way from the days of the barber surgeons who would ride into town and village in their wagons. Locals in the most acute pain would reluctantly submit to their ministrations, while curious on-lookers observed, horrified, the screams and the flow of blood. The establishment of apprenticed teaching and finally degrees in dental surgery transformed these itinerant opportunists into respected professionals with the title of Doctor!

How well respected? Well the answer was greatly respected and trusted. But a recent Gallup poll shows that while we are still up there with the Pharmacists who still rank number one by the way, we have dropped to fifth place as the most trusted of professionals.

We each have a responsibility not only to our patients, but also to our profession to maintain the highest standards of care, and to communicate honestly at all times. The shadow of our former status lurks there ready to haunt us, and conflicting opinions about just what constitutes "good care" is starting to dog all of our lives.

Kenneth Jacobs wrote a brilliant editorial about the blurring of the lines when we consider dental sub-

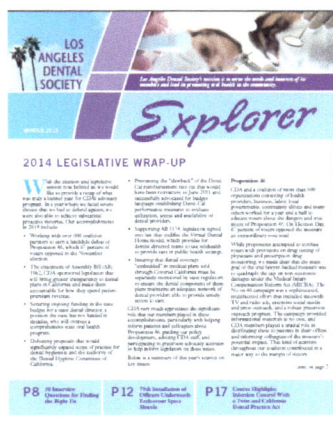

Winter 2015

specialties. Our concern about misrepresentation must extend to being willing to confront our colleagues who appear to make claims that their service is superior to their peers because of their particular focus on one cute little bon bon at the side of the ecclesiastical plate of accepted dental treatments.

Advertising used to be considered unethical for dentists. In fact I distinctly remember that in my Jurisprudence classes we were admonished never to claim that one's services were better than another's. Recounting the words of Hippocrates, allbeit mistakenly, one should "First do no harm". In these days of the internet and the ever increasing battles for cyber citations to boost buoyancy, we have lost sight of judgement in the boldness of our claims. Furthermore, we encourage our patients to write the most fabulous reviews in which they tout the benefits of treatments, and we give accent to allowing their comments to be published. This is a self aggrandizement which amounts to advertising. We are judged by what the public reads about, and they are judging us harshly.

At a time when the competition is offering implants for $398 on billboards on public streets we have reason for concern.

THE OLDEST PROFESSION...

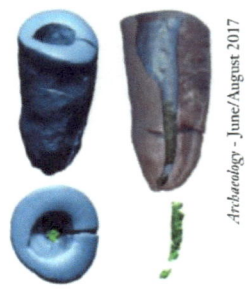

They say that necessity is the mother of invention, and it took an inordinate amount of inventiveness to come up with the skills to provide dental care and make it the profession we are now all so proud to practice.

You do not have to be a historical scholar to have some opinion about to what the title of this chapter might refer. But you may also be surprised. One old profession certainly referenced in Genesis 38:14-26 is the Biblical story of Judah and Tamar a story set around 1010–970 BC. Sumerian records predate that back at 2400 BC with the earliest recorded mention of similar professional activity.

However in the July/August 2017 edition of *Archaeology*, Marley Brown references a different profession - closer to our hearts, which was ostensibly in full swing 11,000 years earlier. Steffano Benazzi of the University of Bologna reports that researchers, working in the hills near Lucca in northern Italy, have found the earliest examples of the practice of filling dental cavities. Two 13,000 year old front teeth that belonged to a late Pleistocene hunter-gatherer, were drilled with a hand tool, decay was removed and the pulp chamber was filled with a "natural antiseptic containing bitumen and vegetal fibers, and hair."

"This new evidence," he wrote," suggests a more sophisticated technology than had been noted from later

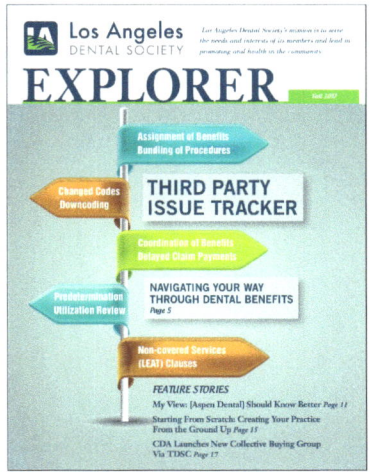
Fall 2017

the evidence. With this revelation we can certainly make the claim that dentistry is demonstrably a very old, if not the oldest profession.

periods, and it is believed to be the first known evidence of human dentistry"

My contention then is that we, as dentists, are practicing the oldest recorded profession in the book.

It can only be imagined in the light of our modern understanding, that from the moment Adam and Eve were turned out of the Garden of Eden, they and their descendants were sentenced to have to look after themselves by themselves. That means attending to the body's needs which inevitably included dental ailments. We are left speculating and examining

NOT THE FIRST... NOR YET THE LAST

We are literally inundated with new products and ideas relating to every conceivable aspect of dental practice. Everything from a "new" design for extraction forceps, surveys on the type of laser "with which you are having success" within your office, to how to promote your web presence better on Bing rather than Google, and of course training courses in Las Vegas which will catapult you to the next level of success in aggressive professional marketing using a new technique.

It is giddying! Yet every time a new idea or concept crosses our desks we have to ask ourselves – is this for me now? Over a hundred years before the first dental college opened its doors in Baltimore, Alexander Pope, the English poet, gave us this great maxim: "Be not the first by whom the new are tried, Nor yet the last to lay the old aside." I remember Peter K. Thomas, that remarkable if bombastic teacher of Gnathology, used to quote this line in his courses. In our bones, we have the sense that, while many of our colleagues are rushing to embrace new technology, and profiting from it, they may also have lowered their critical standard and are not really offering better care.

Really, it is all about the standard of care. We still see and replace silver fillings, asking ourselves who placed these restorations, when we personally may not have inserted an alloy since 1977. By the same token, the gold onlay, so long touted as the premiere restoration, seems to be infrequently placed

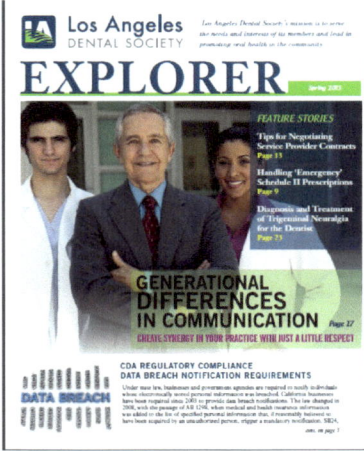

Spring 2015

today in the face of demand for the "white" alternatives. Is the gold onlay going the way of the gold foil? There is a pressure upon each of us to try new products or ideas. It comes in the form of compelling arguments provided by a sophisticated and well funded sales force. They are only too pleased to acquaint us with what we did not yet know, which our patients come into our offices and ask us about. You know, questions like, "Can you fit me with the Zirconium non-metal implants, because I don't want metal in my body?" They have read about it on the Internet or in a popular magazine. Then, of course, there is the elaborate promotional material on the latest one-step bonding agent which will shave thirty seconds off the time it takes to place a filling. We, on the other hand, have yet to be instructed by a reliable academy on whether such additions to our armory of abilities are really efficacious. We have a professional responsibility to be cautious in adopting the "new" while maintaining a respect for the tried and true.

[1] Alexander Pope, An Essay on Criticism, 1711

CAPITALIZING ON CURRENT NEWS

For a dentist making sure that you are getting your share of the pie requires active involvement in social media. You can not get away from the fact that it really matters. That mean that you need to be up to date with news that relates to our discipline.

Recently there has been a spate of questions about the relevance and value of flossing. Can you believe it? This is due greatly to the farcical new criticism of evidence for the value of flossing in helping to preserve your dental health. It is as ridiculous as so many other current issues which deny the obvious and fly in the face of good judgement.

The Associated Press' recent announcement, and the publication the article by Ray Ellen Bitchell on National Public Radio that there is no evidence of the value of

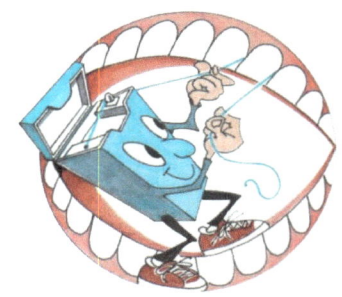

flossing is not to be construed as a reversal of the 1979 edict that we should all floss the teeth we want to keep. The only truth in the report is that they have not conducted long enough clinical trials.

We should all be prepared to answer such questions, and could capitalize on it as Dr. Steven Glassman of New York has when he stated the case clearly on CBS (http://www.cbsnews.com/news/a-big-problem-with-flossing/)

"that the suggestion that we need not floss is a serious mistake, and that neglecting

the spaces between the teeth causes gum disease, decay between the teeth and predisposes you to potential heart attacks. The American Dental Association has not changed its position on the appropriate incorporation of flossing as a regular part of proper oral health care."

By Googling the subject you will be able to find the links and a rebuttal which you can share on your professional facebook page and on LinkedIn, and thereby establish yourself as an active expert in touch with the modern day concerns. You can also tweet about it and add your comments all of which will increase the number of online citations you have which in turn will boost your web presence.

In her 1798 letter to Admiral Lord Nelson, shortly before he left for the battle of the Nile, Lady Hamilton wrote, "Don't forget to pack your dental twine dear!" Nelson returned victorious though minus an arm and many of his teeth. Clearly the upper echelons of society knew, even then, the value of using fine string to clean between the teeth. Everyone should now be flossing.

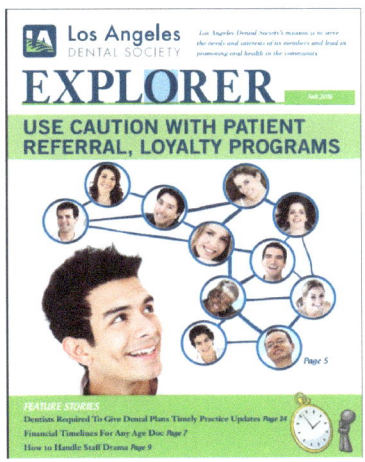

Fall 2016

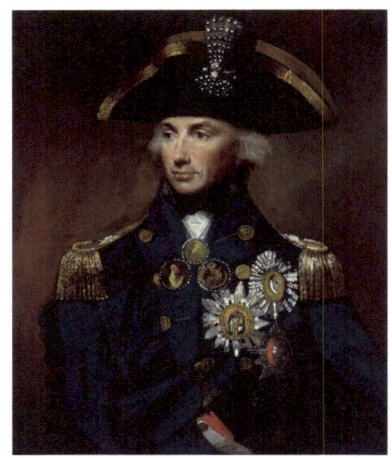

Admiral Lord Nelson Public Domain

Nelson's Floss

Admiral Lord Nelson
Before he sailed to war
Got a letter delivered
From his paramour.
From London it arrived at
Lady Hamilton's behest,
That letter came by carriage
With the Admiral's chest.

Nelson read his letter
He held it with the left,
The right arm it was missing
At Tenerife bereft.
One sentence implored
Our admiral of the line
"Please do not forget, dear,
To pack your dental twine."

The lesson for the taking,
Should you be at a loss
Is that even early on
The best knew they should floss.
'Tho the admiral's dilemma
Might cause you alarm,
Because it's nigh impossible
With only but one arm.

FINAL IMPRESSIONS - THE END OF AN ERA?

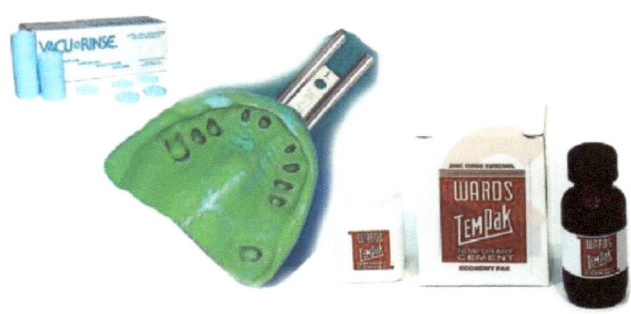

"Sorry we don't carry that any more!" said our representative at Patterson Dental. That was the answer that really got my attention. Suddenly I was rummaging around in the jumble of files which so untidily fill up my mind remembering Tempak, the best temporary filling material ever, and the daisy cup for Vacu Rinse which replaced my cuspidor in 1976.

"We don't have hydrocolloid impression material any more, we can't get it." What they meant was, *"nobody orders that any more Doctor McLeod, you are an old dinosaur!"*

I called Dux and was informed that they had four boxes of heavy bodied tubes and a few hundred cartriloids left, and would I like them. After that it would be over.

Hydrocolloid impression material has been the gold standard for restorative dentistry since Morris Thompson consolidated the technique in the 1950's. By 1974 when I entered USC dental school it was the material of choice for anyone wanting to get really accurate impressions for fine restorations, particularly in gold. Subsequently we as a profession embraced rubber-base and then the new poly vinyl siloxane materials which moved forward in preeminence and slowly superceded the use of hydrocolloid by all but a small cadre of enthusiasts. Now the demand for the seaweed agar is so small that it is being dropped from the catalogues.

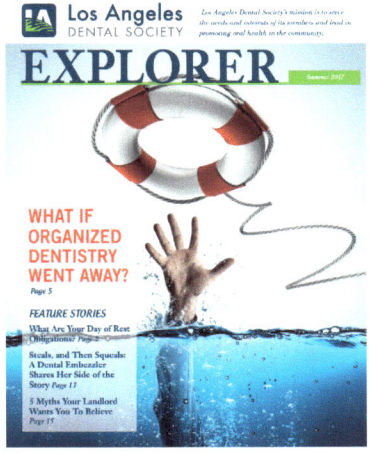

Summer 2017

Overshadowing all of this is the pressure to use digital light impression technology. Even the bite registration can now be indexed using an algorithm that manipulates the data from the light impression files. Today nearly every porcelain or zirconium crown has a base that is carved by a CADCAM system which means that even if you are taking a physical impression it is at least one step removed from the original. So we are actually being forced to change yet again.

This discontinuation of agar comes hand in hand with the introduction of optical impressions. One might compare this with the introduction of digital photography and x-ray imaging. How many of us now still use photographic emulsion for pictures or x-rays? The answer will be the same about impression materials all too soon. My question is are we exchanging quality for convenience?

IS DIGITAL BETTER ?
IS NEW BETTER?

The other day, while driving to my office, dodging the major part of Sunset Boulevard to avoid just seeing the images on the billboards - they can be so sinful - while coming up Hollaway, I saw these graffiti angels.

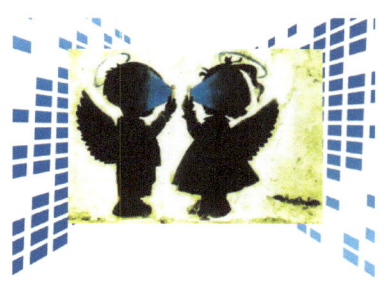

What an interesting juxta-position. There, ahead of me was the site of Tower Records being given a retro facelift with the old original colors back in their former glory because this throwback is popular, liked, even better than the new look. To my side, I flashed on the angels, also flashing selfies or staring in isolation at the all monopolizing cell phones. No longer paying attention to one another.

It hit me that all that is new is not necessarily better. Oh you might say, Dr. McLeod, that is because you are just stuck on gold onlays and are not willing to surrender to the modern changes. That is not entirely true. I do lots of porcelain. It is that I see us all being rushed into digital impressions and budget dentistry, with corporate managers wooing the market so that they can get their share of the cream of the profits on the backs of us clinicians. We will be relieved of our managerial nightmares at the cost of clinical freedom.

I ask myself, "Is digital really better?" The answer is, of course, when used correctly with good clinical judgement, we can incor-porate modern treatment modalities and continue to offer our patients the highest standards of care. This, in an increasingly competitive market, is, of course, the only way to succeed. We must all take responsibility to continually evaluate the new and support one another with meaningful dialogue as each change comes along.

When you consider Wilfred Fish's treatise on dentures and how the surfaces are designed, it is hard to conceive that a light impression can facilitate the model-less carving of a denture base from a solid block of acrylic.

We go from strength to strength by continually striving to rationalize accepting the ever changing world of modern dentistry. We don't want to lose our focus on the bigger picture by being totally self absorbed like those angels.

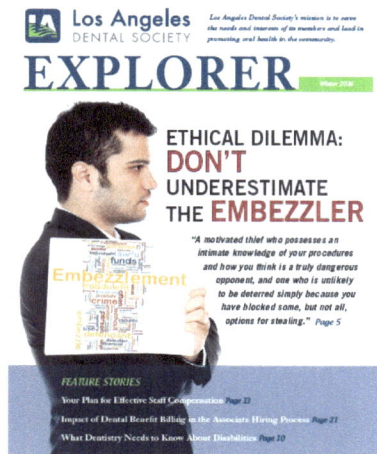

Winter 2016

DON'T RUSH TO BRUSH

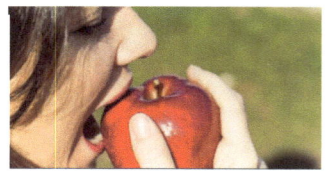

The advantage of being editor of a professional newsletter with a friendly supportive staff is that one's pet peeves can get an airing.

It has been fun to define "Doctor", to express the benefits of the old and the new in dental ideas, to focus on what it takes to upgrade our practices, and to consider our susceptibility to give in to market pressures to adopt "technology" that may not ultimately be efficacious. In my last editorial we considered the possible detriments and benefits of the digital revolution and how they impact dental practice.

While on my high horse, I thought it would be valuable to look backwards and consider that old maxim "*brush after meals*". It turns out that we should not *"rush to brush"*.

Recent research from the University of Adelaide in South Australia[1] on tooth erosion shows that the old advice to "brush your teeth right after a meal" is not correct after all. In fact, we should educate our patients to wait to brush for at least one and a half to two hours after eating because exposure to acidic foods and drinks etches our teeth.

Immediately after biting into fruit, especially a lemon, you notice that the teeth feel rough. What is that rough-ness? The answer is, it is the exposed protein matrix that supports the crystals of the enamel sticking out from the etched surface of the outer part of the tooth that makes it feel rough. Two hours later how does it feel? Smooth again, right?. The saliva in your mouth is a super saturated solution of calcium salts. It actually reconstitutes the external layer of the tooth. If you eat something that's acidic and you immediately go and brush your teeth you damage the protein matrix and eliminate the reconstitution or recrystalization of the outermost part of the tooth. If you brush vigorously immediately after every meal, slowly but surely, you'll be damaging your teeth.[2]

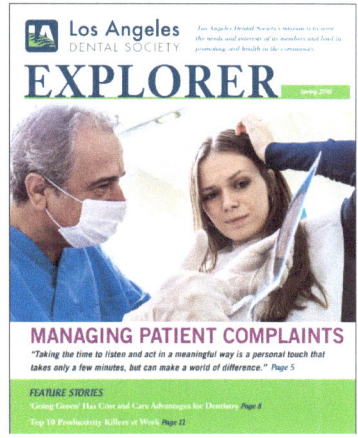

Spring 2016

Don't Rush To Brush[3]

Have you ever bitten into a lemon
And noticed how rough each tooth grows?
Well, they have been etched
And their protein matrix,
Where enamel's dissolved, is exposed.

But check your teeth two hours later
The feeling of roughness is gone,
Your saliva you see
Quite miraculously
Grows the crystals back all on its own.

A lot of our foods are acidic,
We like that it gives them a "bite",
But the protein's exposed
On which enamel grows,
And brushing that off isn't right.

So don't rush to brush after eating.
If you must brush then do it before,
They've been teaching us wrong
For ever so long,
And we shouldn't do that any more.

We used to say brush after eating,
Which would ruin the lingering flavor
The reason they grieve,
Was the food that you leave?
On your teeth does the germs a big favor.

Enjoy your food while you can taste it,
Take time to relax when you're done.
Don't rush to brush
And make all that fuss,
It isn't right and it's not fun.

1. http://www.washingtonsblog.com/2014/01/don't-brush-eating-acidic-food.html

2. http://smallbusinesstrendsetters.com/beverly-hills-dentist-dr-neil-mcleod-says-to-preserve-tooth-enamel-don't-rush-to-brush/

3. http://www.amazon.com/Dental-Ditties-Neil-Stewart-McLeod/dp/1517252504/ref=sr_1_1?ie=UTF8&qid=1449599915&sr=8-1&keywords=Neil+Stewart+McLeod+Poetry

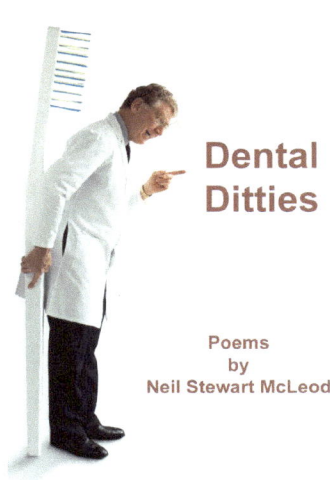

'GIVING IN TO MARKET PRESSURE

Trying to incorporate progressive innovations into our practices is, on the face of it, a good thing. How else will we advance as a profession? I remember what a boon it was when the Borden high speed handpiece was introduced in the late 1960's, and when fiberoptics were put into the Midwest Quietair in 1976. These were and remain great advances in our ability to provide quality care for our patients.

There are other ideas which are marketed to us which we feel equally encouraged to take up and latch onto in an ever increasingly competitive race for market share. Pausing to reflect upon some previous examples will help us to temper our impetuosity and possibly slow us from adopting nebulous innovation. In casting my eye backward, the Waterpik controversy and the Atridox/Arestin regimes come to mind. The former does not remove plaque, and one wonders how the Teledyne company has managed to persuade millions of Americans to use this ineffective product. The later antibiotic therapy does not reduce periodontal pockets, well, not more than 0.5mm, which is completely insignificant for those for whom this treatment was prescribed, with pockets over 4 and 5 millimeters. More recently we have had the cancer screening kits with their fluorescent dyes and the test strips for an array of predispositions, none of which outdo the human eye and the prescription for regular brushing and flossing and checkups, and all of which are extraordinarily expensive. While practice efficiency experts recommend marketing such additions to boost "production," I can't help having to admit that I felt slimy even considering it.

Looking to the present, and setting aside digital impressions and instant CAD CAM crowns and inlays, which I do not want to frown on today, I would like to focus on social media and paying for favorable cyber-presence. If you have not been approached with a barrage of e-mails from a litany of companies touting their expertise at boosting your practice visibility, then you must be off the map somewhere. There is no doubt about it, the internet has completely changed the way patients look for and determine where they are going to receive care. We, as a profession, are constantly being told that we have to subscribe to this or that new service in order to be found on the internet.

The truth is that having numerous accurate concordant citations will enhance the way your practice appears in the search results. However, perhaps the most important thing you can do is to have lots of good reviews on the various sites where they are displayed. Google plus, CitiSearch, Yelp, Angie's List, Healthgrades and many others are good places to encourage reviewers to comment.

Which brings me to the point I wanted to make. Be cautious about signing contracts to pay to enhance your web presence. Simply having new threads posted, and artificially engaging in forums on social media sites can look fake and be costly. On the other hand, you have to cross Yelp management's palm with silver if you want to keep all your good reviews up and suppress the negative which is so unethical.

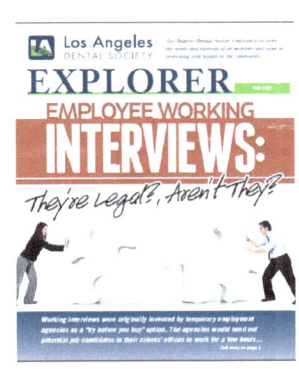

Fall 2015

ARE YOU MAKING THE upGRADE?

Like it or not we are all still expected to make the grade. That does not just mean taking refresher courses or knowing the latest innovations that are coming down the pipeline and how and when to integrate them into our practices. Basic IT (information technology) is now going through a major upheaval that is effecting us all.

Let us consider for a moment the withdrawal of support for Windows XP, the work horse that we have been using for fourteen years. There is no option, all our programs need to be upgraded to work on the new Windows 7 platform. The computer in each work station must be networked to the server so that the images we capture, both digital x-rays and intraoral camera shots, can be seamlessly integrated into the data management program. They all have to be changed, and then of course, backed up both locally and to "the cloud" so that we do not run the risk of losing data. Oh, and let's not forget being transferred in a HIPAA compliant format! Well, that's a lot to bite off in one go. What gets interesting and discouraging is finding out that our favorite intraoral camera does not work on the new Microsoft program. If you liked Accucam, with its foot control capture, variable focal length and the ability to turn off the illumination at will so that you can demonstrate fiber-optically transilluminated fractures, then the new USB connected cameras can be really disappointing. There is a way to pay for all this new stuff, and that is by taking advantage of the new VOIP (Voice Over Internet

Protocol) telephone and high-speed internet connections. Reduce the number of phone lines coming into your office to just one, but keep your numbers and fax line. Cutting costs here can make a big difference. Perhaps the most important place to make the grade is online with your web presence - personal cyber-buoyancy (yes you may use the term*). We all have to have dynamic and mobile websites so that searchers can find us on line. Our websites need to be updated regularly so that the search engine crawlers (now called spiders) count ours as newly updated sites. We also need to have videos about what we do best so that our patients know about our expertise.

Finally, we need to make the grade by having good reviews online from our satisfied patients. This part of our social network reputation is essential. No matter where your referrals come from, people are going to go online and look you up. They look up everything else, and they are going to check

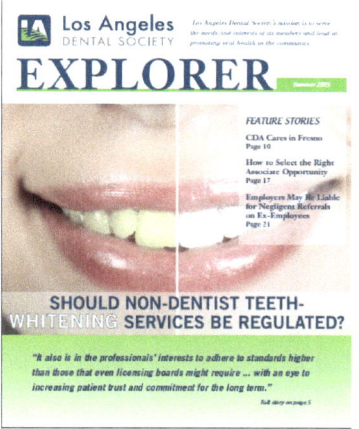

Summer 2015

you out too. If you do not have a good web presence they will automatically know that "something is wrong". The reviews about you must be plentiful and flattering. Otherwise, you will become relegated to the sixth or ninth or twenty seventh page on Google, where nobody goes to find a dentist!

So we are all past the point where we ask ourselves "Do I need a website?". Web presence is essential we are all agreed, it is the crown of your marketing tools; and yes it needs to be dynamic so we can change it at will, and it must be mobile friendly so that we show up on phones and tablets. But... there is more to it than that! A lot of us do not own our own website or it's content, and the moment we stop paying our monthly fee the site will be taken down. Furthermore, we are blocked from discovering where traffic came from and what was looked at that worked as far as serving the searchers on line is concerned.

It is becoming increasingly important to have a fresh looking website, and one which has been updated recently using information which analysis shows is likely to have impact and draw searchers to seek for your services. The cookie cutter sites, like those of Prosites and Officite while they are dynamic and can be updated, prevent you from using analytical tools to assess how your site performed. What's more, you don't own it. There is a constant flow of dollars from you pocket just to stay on line.

There is a growing trend to take advantage of the opportunity to build your own web site, that you can edit, that is mobile friendly, and which allows you to analyze the traffic. Big players want to get into this business and now is a very good time to be looking seriously at "remaking that crown".

* "Enhancing the online presence of a dental practice," Neil S. McLeod – JPD, April 2012

A BRAIN WAVE

EDITOR'S CORNER
By Neil McLeod, BDS, LDS, RCS, DDS

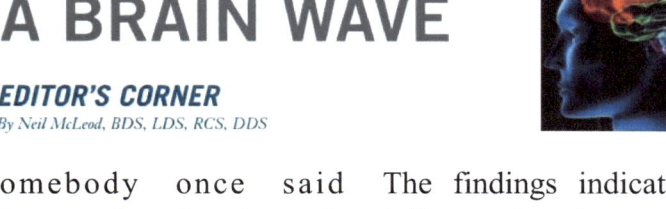

Somebody once said "Preservation of tooth equals preservation of youth", it was one of my professors and I have been quoting the line ever since. It seems like a useful maxim that members of our profession can rattle off to good effect when trying to motivate patients to be compliant with our home care recommendations. The fact is though, it was never more true, so I encourage you all to latch on and quote it.

A few weeks ago I attended a lecture given by Dr. Marc Milstein, Lecturer and Scientist at UCLA. His subject, "Key Insights Into Protecting Your Brain." It was a fascinating talk. It linked oral health clearly with brain health, and in a number of ways. First of all, new research has clearly connected inflammation in the mouth to heart disease and now brain disease.

The findings indicate that inflammation increases the likelihood of developing dementia. Dr. Milstein surprised us all by stating that the brain literally shrinks to 40% of its volume during deep sleep, and that in doing so it flushes out a wave of fluid from between the axons into the cerebrospinal fluid which then drains into venous capturing through a duct opening into the neck. He explained that inflammation interferes with this process. He also stressed that if some one is showing signs of dementia, that first question that should be asked is "Are they suffering from sleep apnea?" The interruption to healthy sleep patterns predisposes our brains to "dementia causing changes".

Well that was good enough for me to justify an even more enthusiastic exhortation to my patients. Not caring for your teeth will cause you to look old, and will actually age your brain. So here is another tool in our kit to encourage our patients to maintain good oral hygiene and do whatever it takes to ensure long regular healthy sleep. That might include using a CPAP, losing weight, exercising, eating better, walking every day, learning something new regularly, and of course brushing and flossing your teeth.

So here is the brain wave, add "the mouth and brain aging" and "gum disease and losing you mind" to your dialogue with patients.

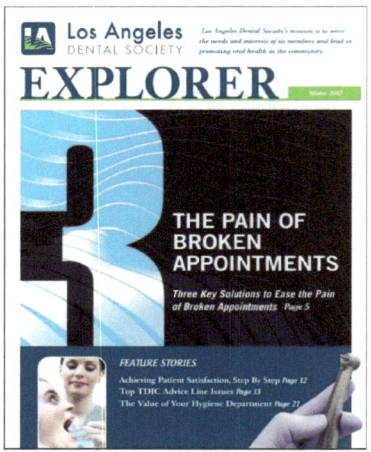

Winter 2017

SAD OR SORRY
DENTAL SERVICE ORGANIZATIONS – A EUPHEMISM

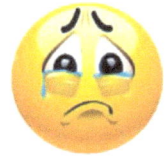

It is axiomatic to accept the maxim that "you get what you pay for". We intuitively understand that quality costs more, and for the services we provide this is certainly true. We are admonished however not to make claims that our treatments are any better than those of our colleagues, after all we certainly do not want anyone to receive second class care.

Dentistry is an art, a combination of skill and training with science and imagination that allows the application of these faculties to relieve our patients pain, and give them a biting chance at life. It is counter intuitive therefore to interpose an insurance company or a corporate manager between the care provider and the patient, and preserve the expectation that the cost of management will not in some way make the service cost more. It does! Both are for profit organizations and if they were not making money they would fold and close up shop.

Insurance companies pitch reduced costs for dental care to a large group, and dish out meager coverage for treatments to those who actually submit a claim. Participating dentists are paid less for the work they do. Dental service organizations (DSO's) purport to market the services of dentists and profess to manage the practices more efficiently. They promote dental care as a brand. Dentists sign up in the hope that they will have more patients driven to seek care in a practice that is run more efficiently. Dental service organizations will increasingly take advantage of regulatory changes which may increase the scope of procedures that midlevel providers (MLPs) may perform. Participating dentists are paid less for the work they do.

Here in Los Angeles as across the country we are still seeing a growth in the number of DSO's; there are now sixty five and counting. Each of them has a strategic concept of the dental marketplace and how best to achieve success. Fundamentally they all try to achieve efficiencies through economies of scale, resulting in a relentless focus on controlling costs of practice operations, and ensuring maximal employee productivity.

We should be concerned about any one who says they can perform the services we provide more efficiently for less money. Any additional layer of management is bound to cut into the resources available to compensate the treatment providers for their services. Dentistry is not cheap and it can not be free. Our concern should not be that they will displace us private practitioners, but for the patients who receive the discounted service for whom we should feel sad, and our unfortunate peers who have made the mistake of signing up with

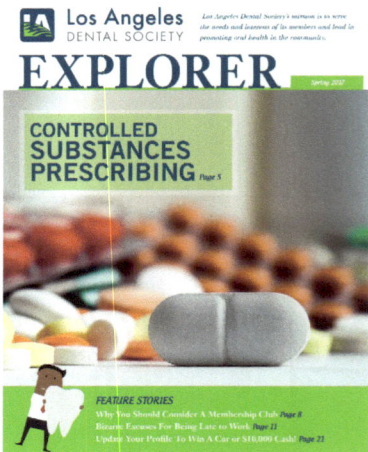

Spring 2017

managed care and now can't wait to get out of their contractual deals. They are feeling very regretful.

In effect these companies are capping and steering, they are receiving compensation for bringing the doctor more treatment opportunities.

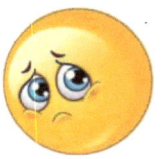

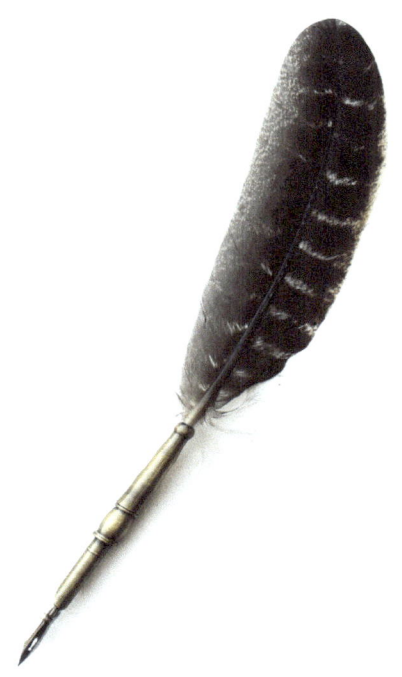

About The Author

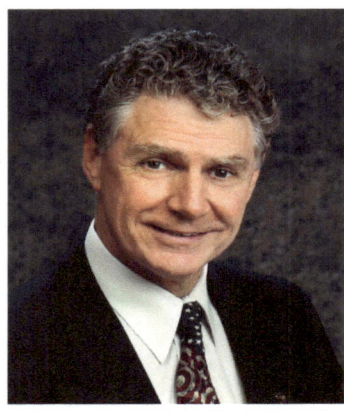

Author - portrait by David Blattel

Neil McLeod was born in Oxford in 1947, while his father attended Merton College. He was raised in Kenya in the 1950's, and received schooling from the Holy Ghost Fathers at Saint Mary's in Nairobi. The family returned to England before the flag was brought down and Kenya gained her Independence. Neil went up to Guy's Hospital to study dentistry and came to America as a Fulbright Scholar to continue his studies at the University of Southern California. Doctor McLeod is past winner of the Los Slamgeles Poetry Slam. He writes a blog spot called *"A Biting Chance"*, where much more of his poetry may be read.

Dr. McLeod is a performing poet who has recited at Highland Games, consulate dinners and Robert Burns Nights for the last 40 years. He is happily married, lives and works in Los Angeles, has three children, and practices as a dentist on Sunset Boulevard. His poem *"The First Thanksgiving"* is an increasingly popular seasonal favorite.

Contact Information

Web: http://www.drneilmcleod.com

e-mail: drneilmcleod@yahoo.com

Blog: abitingchance.blogspot.com

Dr. McLeod will willingly entertain requests to share his work with permission.